Hercules' Sexual Stamina

' Sexual Stamina The Complete Guide to Lasting Longer in Bed Like a God

Dr. Steve JC

Publication date: September 10, 2023

The information provided in this book is intended for educational and informational purposes only. They do not in any way replace medical or professional advice. The author and publisher assume no responsibility for incorrect or inappropriate use of information contained in this book. It is strongly recommended that you consult a qualified healthcare professional or therapist with any medical or sexual questions.

Content

- Presentation of the importance of sexual performance and endurance in bed.
- Justification of the need for a comprehensive guide on the subject.
- Overview of the main ideas and strategies covered in the book.

Chapter 1: Understanding Sexual Stamina

- Definition of sexual stamina.
- Common myths about sexual stamina.
- The importance of endurance for sexual satisfaction.

Chapter 2: Factors Affecting Sexual Stamina

- Physiological factors.
- Psychological factors.
- Relational factors.
- Factors linked to lifestyle.

Chapter 3: The Importance of Communication

- Communication with your partner.
- Communication with a health professional.
- The importance of openness and mutual understanding.

Chapter 4: Stress and Performance Management Techniques

- La relaxation.
- Meditation.
- Breathing.
- Physical exercise.

Chapter 5: Practicing the Stop-Restart Technique

- Explanation of the technique.
- How to practice it effectively.
- The advantages of the technique.

Chapter 6: Pelvic Floor Strengthening Exercises

- The importance of the pelvic floor.
- Strengthening exercises.
- Benefits for sexual stamina.

Chapter 7: Diet and Supplements for Sexual Stamina

- Foods beneficial for endurance.
- Supplements that can help.
- The effects of alcohol, tobacco and drugs on endurance.

Chapter 8: Tips for a Fulfilling Sex Life

- The importance of variety.
- Sexual exploration with your partner.
- The importance of foreplay.

Chapter 9: When to Consult a Professional

- Signs indicating that it is time to consult.
- How to find a trusted professional.

Chapter 10: Summary and Future Outlook

- Summary of main strategies and techniques.
- Encouragement to pursue a fulfilling and healthy sex life.

Conclusion

- Reminder of the importance of sexual endurance.
- Encouragement to put the advice in the book into practice.
- Recognition of readers for their interest.

Introduction

Sexuality is an essential part of our lives, an expression of love, passion and connection between partners. When this experience is fulfilling and satisfying, it can strengthen intimate bonds and bring a sense of well-being to all aspects of our existence. However, there is no denying that sexual performance, and specifically stamina in bed, is often a source of concern for many people.

Sexual stamina, the ability to maintain satisfying sexual intercourse for an extended period of time, is a key component of fulfilling sexuality. Yet it is a subject shrouded in mystery, misunderstanding and sometimes even shame. It's time to break down these barriers and openly explore this crucial area of our intimate lives.

Why a Complete Guide to Sexual Stamina?

This book, "Hercules Sexual Stamina: The Complete Guide to Lasting Longer in Bed Like a God", aims to demystify sexual stamina, provide accurate information and help individuals improve their performance at bed. You don't have to be a god or goddess to live a fulfilling sex life. You only need knowledge, confidence and a few proven techniques.

Our modern society is inundated with conflicting advice, miracle products, and unrealistic expectations when it comes to sexuality. It's time to separate myth from reality and take control of your sex life. This guide will help you understand the factors that influence your sexual stamina, learn practical techniques to improve your performance, and foster open communication with your partner.

Overview of key ideas and strategies

Throughout the pages of this book, we will explore in detail the physiological, psychological, relational and lifestyle factors that influence your sexual stamina. You'll discover practical tips on stress management, communicating with your partner, stop-start techniques, pelvic floor strengthening exercises, the importance of diet and supplements, and much more. other strategies to improve your endurance in bed.

We will also emphasize the importance of living a fulfilling sex life, rich in variety, exploration and foreplay. Finally, we will discuss when it is appropriate to consult a sexual health professional, if necessary.

This book is intended to give you the knowledge and tools you need to achieve better sexual stamina and greater satisfaction in your intimate life. It's time to take charge of your sexuality and live a fulfilling experience, full of confidence and pleasure. Are you ready to embark on this journey to better sexual performance? So, let's get started.

Chapter 1: Understanding Sexual Stamina

Sexual stamina is a complex and often misunderstood area of human sexuality. However, it plays an essential role in sexual satisfaction and general well-being. In this first chapter, we'll dive deep to understand what sexual stamina really is, why it's important, and how it can influence our intimate experience.

Definition of Sexual Stamina

Sexual stamina is an individual's ability to maintain satisfactory sexual activity for an extended period of time. This definition goes well beyond simply being able to last longer in bed, as it encompasses a range of components that contribute to a fulfilling sexual experience. It is essential to understand that sexual stamina is not limited to physical performance, but is also linked to physiological, psychological, relational and lifestyle aspects.

Common Myths About Sexual Stamina

One of the major obstacles to understanding sexual stamina is the proliferation of myths and misconceptions. One of the most common myths is that sexual stamina is primarily about physical performance. Many people wrongly believe that genital size, virility or physical strength are the key factors for having good sexual stamina. However, this belief is erroneous. Sexual stamina is about understanding your own body, managing emotions, and communicating with your partner.

Another common myth is that sexual stamina is innate, that one is born with a special stamina and that nothing can be done to improve it. This is a daunting idea for many people who want to improve their endurance. The truth is that, like any skill, sexual stamina can be developed and improved with time, practice and knowledge.

The Importance of Stamina for Sexual Satisfaction

Why is sexual stamina important? The answer is simple: it plays a crucial role in sexual satisfaction. Increased endurance allows you to prolong sexual pleasure and further explore the pleasures shared with your partner. It allows us to create richer and more fulfilling intimate experiences.

Sexual endurance goes beyond simply prolonging the sexual act. It encompasses the ability to maintain sexual arousal, delay ejaculation (in the case of men), experience pleasure throughout the sexual experience, and be fully present in the moment. This means that sexual stamina is essential to achieving orgasm satisfactorily, for both men and women.

Improved sexual stamina also promotes a better emotional connection with the partner. Couples who can share longer, more satisfying intimate moments are often more in harmony and closer to each other.

In summary, this first chapter laid the foundation for our exploration of sexual stamina. We've clarified its definition, debunked the myths surrounding it, and highlighted its importance for a satisfying sex life. Sexual stamina is not a gift reserved for a privileged few, but a skill that everyone can develop. In the following chapters, we'll dive deeper into the factors that influence sexual stamina and look at practical techniques for improving it. It's time to demystify this topic further and discover how you can become the master of your own sexual stamina.

Chapter 2: Factors Affecting Sexual Stamina

Sexual stamina isn't just a matter of physical strength or willpower. It is influenced by a multitude of factors that interact to create a sexual experience unique to each individual. In this chapter, we will explore in detail the factors that affect sexual stamina, whether physiological, psychological, relational or lifestyle.

Physiological Factors

Physiological aspects play a central role in sexual stamina. Understanding how your body works is essential to improving your endurance. Here are some of the key physiological factors:

1. **The nervous system and ejaculation** : In the case of men, the nervous system has a significant impact on premature ejaculation. Hypersensitivity of the glans, for example, can lead to rapid ejaculation. Understanding how to regulate nerve stimulation can help delay ejaculation.

2. **The circulatory system** : Healthy blood circulation is essential for maintaining an erection

and prolonging sexual activity. Circulation problems can lead to difficulty maintaining an erection or maintaining sexual pleasure.

3. Hormones : Hormones play an essential role in regulating sexual function. Unbalanced hormone levels can affect libido, arousal and sexual performance.

4. The musculature : The pelvic floor muscles are directly involved in sexual endurance. Exercises to strengthen these muscles can help improve control over ejaculation.

Psychological Factors

Psychology also plays a major role in sexual stamina. Emotions, self-confidence and mental state can have a significant impact on sexual performance. Here are some of the psychological factors that come into play:

1. Sexual anxiety : Sexual performance anxiety can cause premature arousal and contribute to premature ejaculation. Learning anxiety management techniques is essential.

2. Self-confidence : Low self-esteem can lead to problems with sexual stamina. Sexual self-confidence is a key element in prolonging sexual pleasure.

3. Focus : Being fully present in the moment is crucial for maintaining sexual arousal and prolonging stamina. Mental distraction can lead to loss of stamina.

4. Past experiences : Past sexual experiences, especially sexual trauma, can have a lasting impact on sexual stamina. Therapy may be needed to resolve these issues.

Relationship Factors

The quality of the relationship between partners plays an essential role in sexual stamina. Open communication, mutual understanding and emotional connection can improve endurance. Here are some of the important relationship factors:

1. Communication : Talking openly about your sexual needs and desires with your partner is essential for a satisfying sex life. Communication can help reduce stress and anxiety related to sex.

2. The emotional connection : Feeling emotionally connected with your partner can improve trust and intimacy, which contributes to better sexual stamina.

3. Mutual understanding : Partners who understand each other's sexual needs and boundaries are more likely to create a positive, lasting sexual experience.

Lifestyle Factors

Finally, lifestyle choices play a significant role in sexual stamina. Healthy lifestyle habits can improve sexual function, while harmful behaviors can compromise it. Here are some of the lifestyle factors:

1. Diet and exercise : A balanced diet and regular exercise promote better blood circulation, which can improve sexual stamina.

2. Sleep : Adequate sleep is essential for sexual function. Fatigue can lead to low libido and endurance problems.

3. Alcohol and substance use : Alcohol and drug abuse can negatively impact sexual function, including stamina.

Ultimately, sexual stamina is influenced by a variety of factors, whether physiological, psychological, relational or lifestyle. Understanding these factors is the first step towards improving your sexual stamina. In the following chapters, we will explore practical techniques for managing these factors and improving your sexual performance. It's time to take control of your sex life and work towards a stamina that will allow you to fully enjoy every intimate moment.

Chapter 3

The Importance of Communication in Sexual Endurance

Communication is a fundamental part of any successful relationship, including the one you have with your sexual partner. In this chapter, we will explore in depth the importance of communication for sexual stamina. We'll look at how open, honest and respectful communication can have a significant impact on the quality of your sex life, while reducing the stress and anxiety that can hinder your performance.

Communication: Foundation of a Fulfilling Sex Life

Communication is key to understanding your partner's needs, wants, and boundaries, as well as expressing your own. It helps create an environment where both partners feel heard, respected and safe to share their sexual fantasies, concerns and expectations.

1. Open the Door to Mutual Understanding

Open communication is the first step in fostering mutual understanding between partners. By talking freely about your desires and preferences, you help your partner better understand what turns you on and what satisfies you. This creates an opportunity to align your mutual expectations and explore new dimensions of intimacy together.

Open communication also helps clear up potential misunderstandings. Often people have preconceived ideas about what their partner wants or doesn't like in bed. By discussing your preferences, you can correct these misunderstandings and avoid embarrassing or frustrating situations.

2. Reduce Stress and Anxiety

Sexual performance anxiety is a common concern for many people. It can cause premature arousal, premature ejaculation or even an inability to maintain an erection. Communication plays a major role in reducing this stress and anxiety.

By sharing your concerns with your partner, you can demystify them. Your partner can reassure you, support you and help you de-escalate the situation. Together, you can find solutions to manage sexual anxiety, whether through relaxation techniques, counseling, or changes to your sexual practices.

3. Create a Space of Trust

Open communication creates a space where both partners feel confident in expressing their needs and boundaries. This promotes a fulfilling sexual relationship, where everyone feels free to explore and experiment without fear of judgment or rejection.

Confidence is essential to maintaining optimal sexual stamina. When you know you can count on your partner's support and understanding, you are more comfortable and relaxed during sexual activity. This allows you to focus on pleasure and satisfaction, rather than worries and doubts.

Communication Techniques for Improved Sexual Stamina

Now that we've established the importance of communication in sexual stamina, let's explore some specific communication techniques that can help you improve your sex life. These techniques will help you better understand your partner, express your needs, and manage sexual anxiety.

1. Active Listening

Active listening is a crucial skill for effective communication. This means being fully present when your partner speaks, listening carefully to what he or she is saying, without interrupting or judging. Active listening helps show your partner that you care about their thoughts and feelings.

When you actively listen, you are able to better understand your partner's needs and wants. This creates a solid foundation for alignment of expectations and for better coordination during sexual activity.

2. Talk about Fantasies

Sexual fantasies are an integral part of human sexuality. Yet many people are hesitant to talk about it with their partner for fear of appearing strange or deviant. Open communication about fantasies can be extremely fulfilling.

Encourage each other to share your deepest, most intimate fantasies. Explain what excites you and what attracts you. You might find that your fantasies come together and you can act out them together, which can greatly improve your sexual stamina.

3. Express Needs and Limitations

It is essential to clearly communicate your sexual needs and limits to your partner. If you have particular preferences, specific erogenous zones, or practices that you want to explore, say so openly. Likewise, if you have boundaries or things you don't want to do, it's important to communicate those as well.

Expressing your needs and boundaries creates a space where you can feel comfortable and respected. This allows you to relax more during sexual activity, knowing that you are on the same page as your partner.

4. Manage Sexual Anxiety Together

If you or your partner suffers from sexual performance anxiety, work together to manage it. Encourage each other to talk about your concerns and experiences. Be understanding and offer unconditional support.

You can also explore techniques for managing sexual anxiety together. Meditation, deep breathing, and relaxation exercises can be effective in reducing stress before and during sexual activity.

Communication as the Foundation of Sexual Endurance

Communication is an essential pillar of sexual stamina. It promotes mutual understanding, reduces stress and anxiety, creates a space of trust and allows you to explore new dimensions of your intimacy together. By using the communication techniques we've explored, you can strengthen the connection with your partner and improve your sexual stamina significantly.

Remember that communication is an ongoing process. The more openly you talk with your partner, the more you strengthen your emotional and sexual connection. Explore your desires, fantasies, and boundaries together, and be willing to adjust your communication as your relationship evolves and your individual needs.

In the next chapter, we'll discuss another essential factor in sexual stamina: self-confidence. You will discover how to develop strong self-confidence, which is a key element in maintaining satisfactory sexual performance. Stay committed to your journey to better sexual stamina, as each step brings you closer to a fulfilling and lasting sex life.

Chapter 4

Stress and Performance Management Techniques

In this chapter, we'll dive deep into stress and performance management techniques, crucial skills for improving sexual stamina. Performance stress and anxiety are common obstacles that can hinder your sexual experience. By understanding and mastering these techniques, you can not only extend your endurance, but also create a more fulfilling and relaxed environment for you and your partner.

1. Deep Breathing: Calm in the Heart of the Storm

Deep breathing is one of the simplest and most effective techniques for managing stress and anxiety. It involves breathing slowly and deeply, focusing on inhalation and exhalation. Here's how it can help you:

has. Reduction of Physical Tension : In times of stress or anxiety, the muscles of the body can become tense. Deep breathing helps relax these muscles, promoting a state of physical relaxation which is conducive to better sexual endurance.

b. Calming of the Spirit : Deep breathing calms the nervous system, thereby reducing anxious thoughts. It allows you to focus on the present moment, rather than on concerns related to performance.

vs. Managing Early Arousal : When you feel yourself getting closer to early arousal, deep breathing can help you slow down and control your sexual response. Take slow, deep breaths to slow the pace of sexual activity.

2. Meditation: The Art of Mindfulness

Meditation is a stress management technique that promotes mindfulness and relaxation. It involves focusing on the present moment, releasing distracting thoughts and deeply relaxing. Here's how meditation can improve your sexual stamina:

has. Overall Stress Reduction : Regular meditation decreases overall stress in your life, which can have a positive impact on your sexual experience. A calmer, less stressed mind is better able to handle the challenges of sexual performance.

b. Sexual Anxiety Control : Meditation teaches you to recognize anxious thoughts and let them pass. This can be particularly helpful for managing sexual performance anxiety.

vs. Increased body awareness : Meditation improves your body awareness, which can help you better perceive your body's signals during sexual activity. This allows you to respond more effectively to physical sensations and adjust your pace to extend endurance.

3. Progressive Relaxation: Relaxing the Muscles and the Mind

Progressive relaxation is a technique that involves deliberately relaxing each muscle group in your body, from head to toe. It can be used to manage stress and anxiety, as well as improve sexual stamina. Here's how it works:

has. Muscle relaxation : By releasing muscle tension, you reduce physical stress that can be associated with sexual anxiety. This allows your body to respond more effectively to sexual stimuli.

b. Concentration on the Body : Progressive relaxation causes you to focus on your body, which strengthens the connection between mind and body. It can improve your body awareness during sexual activity.

vs. Reduction of Emotional Tension : Progressive relaxation also promotes emotional relaxation. By releasing emotional tension, you are better able to fully engage in the sexual experience without being hindered by stress or anxiety.

4. Positive Visualization: Creating a Satisfying Scenario

Positive visualization is a powerful technique that involves imagining satisfying sexual scenarios. It can be used to boost self-confidence, reduce stress and anxiety, and prolong endurance. Here's how it can help you:

has. Strengthening Self-Confidence : Visualizing successful sexual scenarios builds your confidence in your sexual abilities. The more confident you are, the less likely you are to experience performance anxiety.

b. Reduction of sexual anxiety : Visualizing positive sexual situations can reduce sexual performance anxiety by creating satisfying mental experiences. This can help you feel more comfortable and relaxed during actual sexual activity.

vs. Prolongation of endurance : Visualizing prolonged sexual activity in your mind can help you maintain a slower pace and prolong endurance. You can imagine moments of break or control when you need them.

Ultimately, stress and performance management techniques are valuable tools for improving your sexual stamina. Deep breathing, meditation, progressive relaxation, and positive visualization can all help reduce stress and anxiety, allowing you to fully enjoy your sex life. By integrating them into your routine, you strengthen your skills to handle performance challenges and create a more relaxed and satisfying intimate environment.

Chapter 5

Practicing the Stop-Restart Technique

The stop-start technique is a proven method for improving sexual stamina by prolonging pleasure and delaying ejaculation. In this chapter, we'll explore this technique in detail, guiding you through the steps to practicing it successfully. By understanding how this method works and incorporating it into your sex life, you will be able to extend your stamina and provide both yourself and your partner with a more satisfying sexual experience.

1. Understand the Shutdown-Restart Technique

The stop-start technique is a behavioral approach that aims to delay ejaculation by controlling sexual arousal. It can be practiced alone or with a partner. Here's how it works:

a. Phase d'excitation : During sexual activity, there is an arousal phase where sexual arousal increases. As arousal increases, you get closer to ejaculation.

b. Point of no return : Before ejaculation, there is a point of no return where it becomes very difficult, if not impossible, to delay ejaculation. This is where the stop-start technique comes into play.

vs. Stop : When you approach the point of no return, you stop sexual activity or stimulation. This may mean stopping movements, temporarily removing the penis from the vagina, or ceasing all stimulation.

d. Reboot : After stopping, you wait a few moments until the excitement subsides slightly. Then you can resume sexual activity or stimulation. This stop-start cycle can be repeated several times during a sexual session.

2. The Advantages of the Stop-Restart Technique

The stop-start technique offers several benefits that help improve sexual stamina:

has. Ejaculation Control : The technique allows you to take control of your ejaculation by learning to recognize your point of no return and delaying it. This allows you to prolong the pleasure for yourself and your partner.

b. Anxiety Reduction : Knowing you have a method to control ejaculation reduces performance anxiety. This makes you feel more comfortable and relaxed during sexual activity.

vs. Sensual Exploration : The stop-start technique encourages a slower, more sensual exploration of intimacy. It promotes a deeper connection between partners, as it requires open communication and mutual understanding of body signals.

d. Practice Solo or Couple : You can practice the technique alone to develop your skills, then integrate it into your sex life as a couple. This allows your partner to actively participate in improving your endurance.

3. Steps to Practice the Stop-Restart Technique

Practicing the stop-start technique can be broken down into simple steps to maximize its effectiveness. Here's how you can implement it successfully:

has. Preparation : Start by making sure you and your partner are in a comfortable, relaxed environment. Open communication is key, so make sure you can talk openly about your concerns and desires.

b. Stimulation initiale : Begin sexual activity normally, focusing on sensations and mutual pleasure. As arousal increases, pay attention to your level of arousal and how close you are to your point of no return.

vs. Stop : When you feel that you are approaching the point of no return, stop or ask your partner to stop the stimulation. Take a few moments to breathe deeply and relax.

d. Reboot : After stopping, wait for the excitement to subside slightly. You can use this time to explore other forms of stimulation, such as caressing, kissing, or erotic communication. Then resume sexual activity or stimulation.

e. Repetition : Repeat the stop-start cycle as many times as necessary to prolong pleasure and delay ejaculation. The more you practice this technique, the more you will be able to recognize and control your point of no return.

f. Communication : Open communication with your partner is essential during this practice. Share your feelings, ask your partner for clues about your arousal level, and listen to their needs and desires.

g. Mutual satisfaction : The goal of the stop-start technique is to create a satisfying sexual experience for both partners. Be sure to consider your partner's needs and desires, and don't hesitate to adjust the practice accordingly.

4. Patience and Perseverance

The stop-start technique requires patience and perseverance. It may take time to master this method and see significant results. So be patient with yourself and with your partner.

5. Integration into Sexual Life

Once you've developed your skills with the stop-start technique, you can integrate it naturally into your sex life to get the most out of it. Here's how you can do it:

5. Integration into Sexual Life

Use During Sex : When you feel ready to incorporate the stop-start technique into your sex, start slowly. You can apply it during sex by identifying your point of no return and using stopping and starting to prolong the pleasure. This method can be especially beneficial if you have a habit of ejaculating quickly. Start with short sessions, then gradually increase the duration as you gain confidence.

Preliminary Practice : Preliminaries provide an excellent opportunity to integrate the stop-start technique. Take your time to explore your partner's body, using sensual caresses and kisses. If you feel the arousal building up quickly, stop momentarily, take a deep breath, and resume when the arousal has subsided. This approach promotes a more emotional and connected sexual experience.

Erotic Games and Fantasy: You can also incorporate the stop-start technique into erotic games and fantasy scenarios with your partner. These games can add an exciting dimension to your sex life while allowing you to practice arousal control.

Open Communication and Consent : Be sure to maintain open communication with your partner throughout the incorporation of the stop-start technique. Ask your partner what works for them and what doesn't. Mutual consent is essential to ensure a positive sexual experience.

Gradual progression : Remember that integrating new sexual techniques can take time. Be patient with yourself and with your partner. Start slowly and work your way up to avoid feeling overwhelmed.

6. Discovering Your Own Preferences

Incorporating the stop-start technique into your sex life can help you better understand your own sexual preferences. You will discover how your body reacts to different forms of stimulation and how you can adjust your pace to prolong the pleasure. This awareness can enrich your sex life in the long run.

7. Communication as the Key to Success

Open communication is essential when incorporating the stop-start technique into your sex life. Pay attention to your partner's signals, listen to their needs and desires, and share yours. The more you communicate, the more you can adjust your practice to maximize pleasure for both of you.

8. Sensual Exploration Continues

Incorporating the stop-start technique into your sex life encourages continued sensual exploration. It leads you to slow down and savor each intimate moment, strengthening the emotional connection with your partner.

Successfully integrating the stop-start technique into your sex life can transform your sexual experience into a fulfilling and satisfying adventure. It offers benefits such as ejaculation control, reduced performance anxiety, and deeper intimacy with your partner. With practice, patience and open communication, you can enrich your sex life and create unforgettable intimate moments for yourself and your partner. Sexual stamina is a valuable skill that allows you to fully enjoy every moment of pleasure.

Chapter 6

Pelvic Floor Strengthening Exercises

Strengthening the pelvic floor is an essential component of improving sexual stamina. In this chapter, we'll explore pelvic floor strengthening exercises in detail, their role in improving sexual stamina, and how to effectively incorporate them into your daily routine. These exercises can bring significant benefits to your sex life, including better ejaculation control, better erections, and greater satisfaction for you and your partner.

1. Understanding the Pelvic Floor

The pelvic floor is a group of muscles located at the base of your pelvis. It supports the pelvic organs, including the bladder, rectum and, in men, the prostate. These muscles play a crucial role in various bodily functions, including urination, defecation, and, of course, sexual function.

2. Role of the Pelvic Floor in Sexual Endurance

The pelvic floor is directly involved in controlling ejaculation and maintaining an erection. Strong pelvic muscles help better control premature ejaculation reflexes by preventing sperm from coming out too quickly. Additionally, they promote optimal blood circulation, which can contribute to firmer erections and better sexual stamina.

3. Pelvic Floor Strengthening Exercises

Pelvic floor strengthening exercises, also called Kegel exercises, are designed to specifically target the pelvic floor muscles. Here's how to make them:

has. Muscle Location : To begin, identify the pelvic floor muscles by practicing stopping the flow of urine when you urinate. The muscles you use to perform this action are the pelvic floor muscles.

b. Position de base : You can do these exercises in any position, whether standing, sitting or lying down. Choose the one that suits you best.

vs. Contraction Technique : Contract your pelvic floor muscles as if trying to stop the flow of urine. Hold the contraction for a few seconds, then release.

d. Reps and Sets : Start by doing 10 contractions, holding each contraction for 5 seconds, then release for 5 seconds. Repeat this exercise 3 times a day. Over time, you can increase the number of contractions and the duration of each contraction.

e. Progression : As you feel stronger, you can add variations to your Kegel exercises, such as quick contractions or contractions held for longer periods of time.

4. Benefits of Pelvic Floor Strengthening Exercises

Pelvic floor strengthening exercises offer many benefits that can improve your sexual stamina:

a. Ejaculation control : Strong pelvic muscles allow you to better control ejaculation by delaying the ejaculatory reflex.

b. Improved erection : Kegel exercises promote optimal blood circulation in the pelvic region, which can contribute to firmer, longer-lasting erections.

vs. More Intense Orgasms : By strengthening the pelvic muscles, you can increase the intensity of orgasm for you and your partner.

d. Reduction of Urinary Leakage Problems : Pelvic floor strengthening exercises can help prevent or reduce urinary leakage problems, which is especially beneficial as we age.

e. Greater sexual sensitivity : Strong pelvic muscles can increase sexual sensitivity, thereby improving your overall sexual experience.

5. Integrating Exercises into Your Daily Routine

To get the full benefit from pelvic floor strengthening exercises, it is important to incorporate them into your daily routine regularly. Here are some tips to help you do this:

has. Create a Routine : Choose specific times of the day to do your Kegel exercises, such as morning, midday and evening. This will help you incorporate them consistently into your routine.

b. Use Reminders : Set reminders on your phone or place visible notes to remind you to do your exercises.

vs. Incorporate into other activities : You can do Kegel exercises while you are sitting at the office, while driving or watching TV. They can be done discreetly.

d. Commitment as a Couple : If you are a couple, consider doing pelvic floor strengthening exercises together. This can strengthen your commitment to your sexual health and create additional bonding.

e. Patience and Consistency : The results of Kegel exercises may take time to appear, so be patient. The key is consistency in practice.

6. Recap

Pelvic floor strengthening exercises are an essential component of improving sexual stamina. They offer many benefits, including better ejaculation control, better erection, and greater sexual satisfaction. By integrating these exercises into your daily routine and practicing them consistently, you can improve your sexual experience and fully enjoy every intimate moment with your partner. Strengthening the pelvic floor is a valuable skill that can improve your sex life in the long run.

Chapter 7

Diet and Supplements for Sexual Stamina

Diet plays an essential role in our physical and mental health, including our sexual performance. In this chapter, we'll explore how a balanced diet and certain supplements can help improve your sexual stamina. Understanding the foods and nutrients that support better sexual function is an important step in optimizing your sex life and overall well-being.

1. Foods That Promote Sexual Stamina

A diet rich in certain nutrients can support better sexual stamina. Here are the types of foods to include in your diet to maximize your performance in bed:

has. Foods rich in antioxidants : Antioxidants, such as vitamins C and E, help maintain healthy blood flow, which is essential for good erections. Citrus fruits, berries, nuts and seeds are good sources of antioxidants.

b. Lean Protein Foods : Protein is important for muscle health, including muscles used during sexual activity. Choose lean proteins like chicken, turkey, fish and legumes.

vs. Foods rich in Omega-3 : Omega-3 fatty acids promote blood circulation, reduce inflammation and contribute to heart health. Oily fish like salmon, walnuts and flax seeds are excellent sources of omega-3.

d. Foods High in Zinc : Zinc is an essential mineral for sperm production and overall sexual health. Oysters, pumpkin seeds and legumes are rich in zinc.

e. Foods Containing Arginine : Arginine is an amino acid that can help improve blood circulation and erection quality. Foods rich in arginine include nuts, seeds, soy and dairy products.

2. Hydration

Adequate hydration is crucial for good sexual health. Water promotes blood circulation, which is essential for a firm erection and good ejaculation control. Make sure you drink enough water throughout the day to stay hydrated.

3. Supplements for Sexual Stamina

In addition to a balanced diet, certain supplements can support your sexual stamina. It is important to note that taking supplements should be done with caution and under the supervision of a healthcare professional. Here are some supplements that may be beneficial:

a. L'Arginine : Arginine is an amino acid that can improve blood circulation, which can contribute to better erections.

b. And Ginseng : Ginseng is an herb that has been linked to improved sexual performance and reduced erectile dysfunction.

c. Le Zinc : Zinc is essential for sexual health and sperm production. Taking zinc supplements can be helpful in cases of deficiency.

d. Omega-3 fatty acids: If you are not consuming enough foods rich in omega-3, fish oil supplements may be considered to promote better blood circulation.

e. Essential vitamins and minerals : Make sure you get enough essential vitamins and minerals in your diet or through supplements if necessary. Nutritional deficiencies can affect sexual health.

4. Foods to Avoid

Just as there are foods that promote sexual stamina, there are also foods to avoid to preserve your sexual health. These include:

has. Excessive alcohol : Excessive alcohol consumption can disrupt sexual function and lead to premature ejaculation.

b. Processed and Fatty Foods : A diet high in processed foods and saturated fats can contribute to clogged arteries and circulation problems, which can affect sexual performance.

vs. Excess sugar : Diets high in sugar can lead to health problems, such as diabetes and obesity, which can negatively impact sexual function.

d. Cigarette : Smoking is linked to problems with blood circulation and cardiovascular health, which can lead to erection problems.

5. Balance and Moderation

The key to a healthy diet for sexual stamina is balance and moderation. Rather than focusing on a specific food, it is important to maintain a balanced and varied overall diet. Avoid extremes and focus on whole, fresh, unprocessed foods.

6. Conclusion

A balanced diet and well-chosen supplements can play an important role in improving sexual stamina. However, it is important to remember that diet is only one aspect of sexual performance. Other factors, such as physical fitness, mental well-being and intimate relationships, also play a vital role. By taking a holistic approach to your sexual health, you can optimize your stamina and fully enjoy every intimate moment with your partner.

Chapter 8

Tips for a Fulfilling Sex Life

A fulfilling sex life is the result of a combination of factors, from communicating with your partner to paying attention to your own well-being. In this chapter we will look at a series of tips that will help you improve and maintain a healthy and fulfilling sex life. These tips cover everything from communication to physical health, so you can enjoy your sex life to the fullest.

1. Open Communication

Communication is the cornerstone of a fulfilling sex life. Paving the way for honest and respectful conversations with your partner is essential. Discuss your wants, needs, limits and fantasies. Mutual understanding builds intimacy and trust, creating an environment conducive to a satisfying sex life.

2. Practice Patience

Patience is a virtue in the bedroom. Don't rush, take the time to explore your partner's body, enjoy foreplay and let yourself be carried away by the present moment. Patience promotes an emotional connection and can help delay ejaculation, which is especially beneficial for men.

3. Attention to Mental Health

Your mental well-being has a direct impact on your sex life. Stress, anxiety, depression and other mental health issues can interfere with your sexual desire and performance. Take care of your mental health by seeking the necessary support, whether through therapy, meditation, or other methods.

4. Maintain Good Physical Health

Good physical health is crucial for a fulfilling sex life. Maintain a balanced diet, exercise regularly to improve blood circulation, and avoid harmful behaviors, such as excessive alcohol consumption and smoking.

5. Avoid Routine

Routine can be the enemy of passion. To spice up your sex life, dare to experiment. Try new positions, locations, or erotic role play. Constant exploration can rekindle the flame of passion.

6. Keep the Romance Alive

Romance and emotional intimacy are essential to maintaining a fulfilling sex life. Plan romantic moments with your partner, like candlelit dinners or romantic getaways. Maintaining an emotional connection strengthens your bond and desire for each other.

7. The Importance of the Foreplay

Foreplay is often overlooked, but it's crucial for a satisfying sex life. Take the time to massage, caress and focus on sensory pleasures before going any further. Foreplay increases arousal and sexual satisfaction.

8. Respect Your Partner's Desires and Boundaries

Respecting your partner's desires and boundaries is essential. Make sure you always obtain mutual consent before pursuing sexual activity. Respect the no's and listen to your partner's verbal and non-verbal cues.

9. Experience Fantasies

Fantasies are a normal part of human sexuality. Share your fantasies with your partner and be open to exploring your partner's. Fantasies can be a source of additional excitement and pleasure.

10. Learn to Deal with Sexual Problems

Sexual problems, such as erectile dysfunction or premature ejaculation, are common and can be treated. See a healthcare professional or sex therapist for help if you're having difficulty. Don't let unresolved sexual issues harm your sex life and relationship.

11. Be Open to Sex Education

Sex education is an ongoing process. Be willing to learn and educate yourself about sexuality. Books, online courses, and discussions with health professionals can help you better understand and improve your sex life.

12. Confidentiality and Discretion

Respect confidentiality and discretion when it comes to your sex life. What happens in the bedroom should be kept private between you and your partner. Mutual trust is essential for a fulfilling sex life.

13. Self-Respect

Self-respect is the basis of a healthy sex life. Have confidence in yourself and your body. Learn to love and accept yourself as you are. Self-respect builds self-confidence and sexual satisfaction.

14. L'Exploration Continue

Sexuality is a continuous journey. Be open to exploring and growing in your sex life. Your wants and needs may change over time, and it's important to adapt your sex life accordingly.

15. Don't forget After-Sex

After-sex is just as important as the sexual act itself. Take time to cuddle, kiss, and connect after sex. This strengthens the emotional connection and prolongs intimacy.

In conclusion, a fulfilling sex life relies on a combination of factors, including communication, mental and physical health, romance, and mutual respect. By putting these tips into practice, you can improve your sex life and create an intimate and satisfying experience with your partner. Remember that every person is unique, and it's important to tailor these tips to your own relationship and personal preferences.

Chapter 9

When to Consult a Professional

A fulfilling sex life can be affected by various problems and challenges, whether physical, emotional or relational. In this chapter, we will discuss the signs and situations in which it is recommended to consult a medical professional or a sex therapist. Professional support can be essential to overcome these obstacles and regain a satisfying sex life.

1. Persistent Erectile Dysfunction

Erectile dysfunction (ED), characterized by the recurrent inability to achieve or maintain an erection sufficient for satisfactory sexual activity, is a common problem among men. If you have persistent erection difficulties, it is essential to consult a healthcare professional. ED may be a sign of an underlying problem, such as cardiovascular disease or hormonal imbalance, that requires proper medical evaluation and treatment.

2. Persistent Premature Ejaculation

Premature ejaculation, characterized by ejaculation that occurs too quickly after the start of sexual activity, can have a significant impact on sexual satisfaction. If you suffer from persistent premature ejaculation, it is recommended to consult a sex therapist or medical professional. Specific ejaculation management techniques and therapies may be helpful in improving ejaculation control.

3. Libido Problems

A significant drop in libido, or sexual desire, may be a sign of underlying issues such as stress, depression, hormonal imbalances, or relationship problems. If your sexual desire is persistently low and this is negatively affecting your sex life, it is a good idea to consult a medical professional or sex therapist. A thorough evaluation can help determine the underlying cause of this problem and develop an appropriate treatment plan.

4. Sexual Satisfaction Problems

If you or your partner regularly have difficulty achieving sexual satisfaction, it may be helpful to see a sex therapist. Problems with sexual satisfaction may be related to emotional problems, relationship conflicts, or communication problems. A sex therapist can help identify obstacles and work with you to overcome them.

5. Communication and Relationship Problems

Conflict, lack of communication or trust issues within a relationship can have a negative impact on sex life. If you and your partner are having trouble communicating or resolving relationship issues that are affecting your sex life, seeing a marriage therapist or relationship counselor may be beneficial. These professionals can help you improve your communication and strengthen your emotional connection.

6. Sexual Trauma or Mental Health Issues

Previous sexual trauma or mental health issues, such as post-traumatic stress disorder (PTSD) or depression, can have a significant impact on sex life. If you have experienced sexual trauma or have mental health issues that affect your sexuality, it is important to see a mental health professional or therapist who specializes in treating these issues.

7. Marital Difficulties or Persistent Conflicts

Marital difficulties, ongoing conflict, or loss of emotional connection within a relationship can lead to sexual problems. If you and your partner are struggling to resolve relationship issues that are affecting your sex life, consider seeing a marriage therapist or relationship counselor. Working on relationship issues can have a positive impact on your sex life.

8. Important Changes in Physical Health

Significant changes in physical health, such as surgery, serious medical problems, or medical treatments, can impact sex life. If you or your partner have experienced significant changes in your physical health that affect your sexuality, consult a healthcare professional to discuss necessary adjustments and available options.

9. Sexual Incompatibility

In some relationships, partners may have different sexual needs and desires which can lead to conflict. If you and your partner are struggling to find common ground when it comes to sexuality and this is causing tension, seeing a sex therapist can help facilitate discussion and find solutions that work for your relationship.

10. The Exploration of Sexuality

Sometimes individuals or couples want to explore new dimensions of their sexuality or learn about alternative sexual practices. If you are considering exploring aspects of sexuality that are unfamiliar to you, consult a sex therapist or sexual health professional for appropriate information, advice and support.

In conclusion, consulting a mental health professional, sex therapist, or relationship counselor can be beneficial in many situations related to sex life. It's important to seek help when persistent problems or complex challenges are affecting your sexual satisfaction. A qualified professional can help you identify underlying issues, develop skills, and find solutions tailored to your personal situation.

Chapter 10

Summary and Future Outlook

In this final chapter of our guide "Hercules' Sexual Endurance: The Complete Guide to Enduring Longer in Bed Like a God", we will recap the main points covered throughout the book and discuss future prospects for your sex life. We hope this guide has provided you with useful information to improve your sexual stamina and sexual satisfaction.

Summary of Key Points

During this guide, we've explored a wide range of topics related to sexual stamina and a fulfilling sex life. Here are the key points to remember:

1. The importance of sexual stamina : We have highlighted the importance of sexual stamina for a satisfying sex life, as well as the many benefits it offers.

2. Understand sexual stamina : Chapter 1 laid the foundation by explaining what sexual stamina is and introducing key concepts.

3. Factors affecting sexual stamina : Chapter 2 examined in detail the physiological, psychological, relational and lifestyle factors that influence sexual stamina.

4. Techniques to improve endurance : We covered various techniques and strategies for improving sexual stamina, including stop-start technique, pelvic floor strengthening exercises, and stress management methods.

5. The importance of communication : Chapter 3 highlighted the importance of open communication and mutual understanding in a fulfilling sexual relationship.

6. Tips for a fulfilling sex life : Chapter 8 offered practical advice for improving your sex life, from patience to handling sexual problems and relationship conflicts.

7. When to consult a professional : Chapter 9 identified situations in which it is recommended to consult a mental health professional, sex therapist, or relationship counselor to resolve sexual or relationship problems.

Future Perspectives for Your Sex Life

Now that you've explored these concepts and techniques, it's time to think about the future of your sex life. Here are some perspectives to consider:

1. Continue to practice : Sexual stamina is a skill that improves with practice. Continue to implement the techniques you have learned to build your endurance.

2. Communication continue : Communication is essential to maintaining a fulfilling sex life. Continue to openly discuss your wants, needs, and boundaries with your partner.

3. Evolution of the relationship : Relationships evolve over time. Be open to changes and developments in your sex life. Explore new fantasies, desires and experiences.

4. Health care : Maintaining good physical and mental health is crucial for your sex life. Continue to take care of your body and mind through a balanced diet, exercise and proper care.

5. The future of sexual research : Sexuality research is constantly evolving, which means new discoveries and techniques may emerge in the future. Stay informed about recent developments in the field of sexuality.

6. Relationship perspectives : Your relationship with your partner may change over time. Be open to adapting and growing together. Continue to work on communication, mutual understanding and mutual satisfaction.

7. Sexual well-being : Remember that sexual well-being is an essential component of your overall well-being. Invest time and energy in your sex life to foster continued satisfaction and fulfillment.

Ultimately, your sex life is an important part of your overall well-being. By using the information and techniques presented in this guide, as well as remaining open to opportunities for learning and growth, you can continue to improve your sexual stamina and fully enjoy every intimate moment with your partner.

We hope this guide has been valuable to you in understanding and improving your sexual stamina. We wish you a fulfilling sex life, filled with pleasure, satisfaction and connection with your partner. Remember that every person is unique, and it's important to tailor these tips to your own experience and personal preferences.

Conclusion

Concluding our journey through "Hercules Sexual Stamina: The Complete Guide to Enduring Longer in Bed Like a God", we would like to reiterate the fundamental importance of sexual stamina in a fulfilling sex life. Sexual stamina is not simply a skill to master, but rather an essential element that can transform your intimate experiences into moments of satisfaction and deep connection with your partner.

We strongly encourage you to put into practice the tips and techniques you have learned throughout this book. Knowledge is the first step, but action is the key to transformation. By actively engaging these methods, communicating openly with your partner, taking care of your physical and mental well-being, you can make significant progress in your sexual stamina.

We would like to express our sincere appreciation to our readers for their interest and engagement in this journey of exploring sexuality and endurance. We hope this guide has been a valuable resource for you, helping you understand the many aspects of sexual stamina and discover how to apply them in your own life.

Always remember that your sex life is unique, just like you are. There is no universal standard of sexual performance, but there is unlimited potential for pleasure, satisfaction and connection when you take the time to cultivate your sexual stamina.

We wish you a fulfilling sex life, rich in intimate moments, complicity with your partner and personal development. Continue to explore, learn and grow, because the journey to exceptional sexual stamina is an ongoing adventure.

Thank you for joining us on this journey. Your success in the field of sexual stamina is our greatest satisfaction.

Here's to your continued sexual fulfillment and a life filled with pleasure and deep connections.

Yours sincerely,

Dr. Steve JC, Sexologue

Thank you for reading this book. I invite you to let your opinions in the comments areas.